PREGNANCY PROBLEMS

COMPLETE

SOLUTIONS

BY SPECIALIST DOCTORS

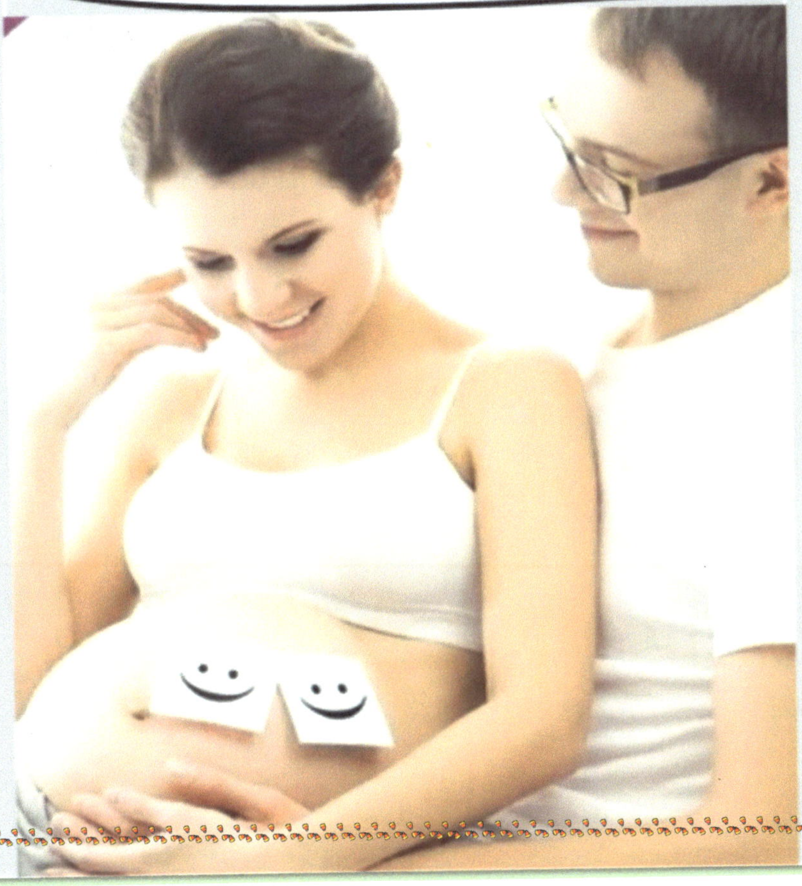

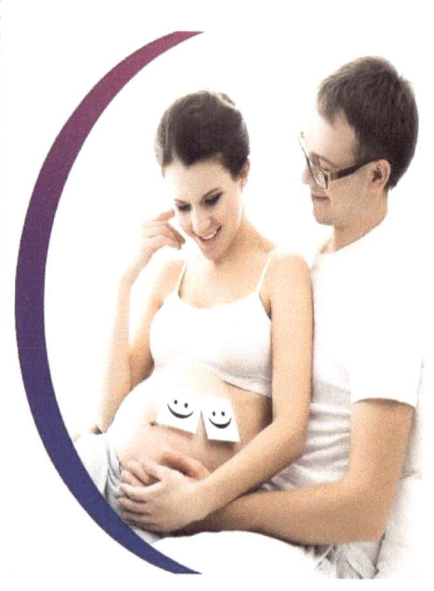

PREGNANCY PROBLEMS AND COMPLETE SOLUTIONS

ABSTRACT

Embark on a journey of hope, knowledge, and empowerment with 'miracle within: navigating pregnancy's path.' leading doctors and specialists, unveils a transformative guide, offering holistic insights and expert advice to embolden couples on their quest for parenthood. Let this book be your beacon of light amidst the struggle

All the best to your journey to getting pregnant!!!

PREFACE

Welcome to pregnancy Welcome to "Pregnancy Problems and Solutions" - a comprehensive guide crafted by specialist doctors aimed at addressing the myriad challenges and concerns that expectant mothers may encounter during the miraculous journey of pregnancy.

Pregnancy is a remarkable period in a woman's life, marked by profound physical, emotional, and psychological changes. While it is a time of great joy and anticipation, it can also bring about various uncertainties and challenges. Understanding and navigating these challenges is crucial for ensuring a safe and healthy pregnancy for both the mother and the baby.

In this book, our team of specialist doctors draws upon their extensive experience and expertise to provide invaluable insights, practical advice, and evidence-based solutions to common pregnancy-related issues. From morning sickness and prenatal care to complications such as gestational diabetes and preeclampsia, we aim to empower expectant mothers with the knowledge and resources they need to make informed decisions and optimize their health and well-being throughout pregnancy.

We recognize that every pregnancy is unique, and individual circumstances may vary. Therefore, while this book offers general guidance, we encourage readers to consult with their healthcare providers for personalized care and advice tailored to their specific needs.

Our ultimate goal is to support expectant mothers in their journey towards a healthy and fulfilling pregnancy, ensuring that they feel empowered, informed, and well-prepared every step of the way.

We sincerely hope that "Pregnancy Problems and Solutions" serves as a valuable companion and trusted resource for expectant mothers, their families, and healthcare professionals alike.

Wishing you a safe, healthy, and joyous pregnancy journey.

TABLE OF CONTENTS :

INTRODUCTION TO PREGNANCY AND ITS CHALLENGES

Pregnancy, the miraculous journey of bringing a new life into this world, is a remarkable and transformative experience for a woman and her family. It marks the beginning of a profound physiological, emotional, and psychological journey, filled with moments of joy, anticipation, and sometimes, challenges.

In this introductory chapter, we delve into the multifaceted nature of pregnancy and explore the various challenges that expecting mothers may encounter along the way. From conception to childbirth, each stage of pregnancy presents its own set of unique circumstances, requiring careful attention and support.

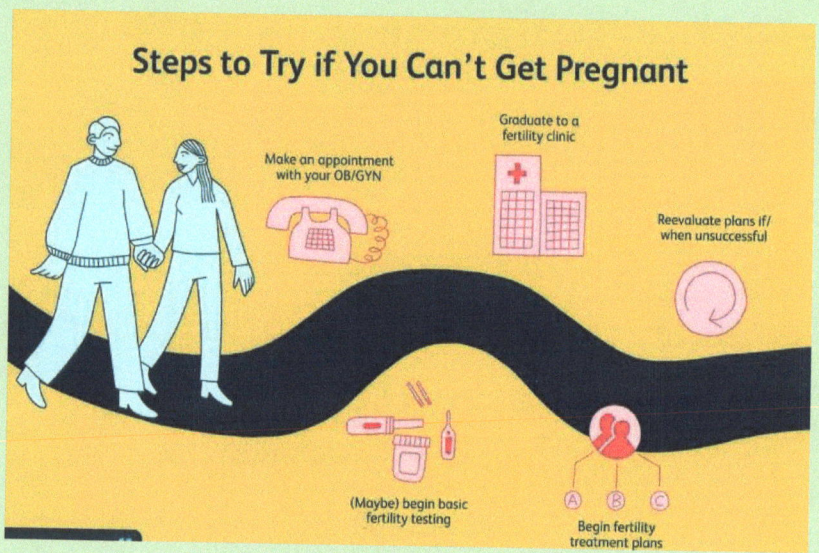

Steps to Try if You Can't Get Pregnant

Make an appointment with your OB/GYN

Graduate to a fertility clinic

Reevaluate plans if/ when unsuccessful

(Maybe) begin basic fertility testing

Begin fertility treatment plans

1. Understanding Pregnancy: Pregnancy, typically lasting around 40 weeks, is divided into three trimesters, each characterized by specific developmental milestones for both the mother and the baby. From the initial stages of conception, where a single cell transforms into a complex organism, to the final moments of labor and delivery, pregnancy is a time of immense growth and change.

2. Physiological Changes: The female body undergoes a series of remarkable physiological adaptations to accommodate the growing fetus. Hormonal fluctuations, changes in blood volume, and alterations in organ function are just a few examples of the intricate processes that occur during pregnancy. Understanding these changes is crucial for ensuring the health and well-being of both mother and baby.

3. Emotional and Psychological Considerations: Pregnancy is not just a physical journey but also an emotional and psychological one. Expectant mothers may experience a wide range of emotions, from excitement and happiness to anxiety and fear. Hormonal fluctuations, coupled with the stress of impending parenthood, can amplify these

feelings. It is essential to address the emotional needs of pregnant women and provide them with the necessary support and resources.

4. Common Challenges During Pregnancy: Despite the beauty and wonder of pregnancy, it is not without its challenges. From morning sickness and fatigue to more serious complications such as gestational diabetes and preeclampsia, expecting mothers may encounter various obstacles along the way. It is imperative for healthcare providers to educate women about these potential challenges and empower them to make informed decisions regarding their prenatal care.

5. Importance of Prenatal Care: Prenatal care plays a critical role in ensuring a healthy

pregnancy outcome. Regular check-ups, screenings, and diagnostic tests allow healthcare providers to monitor the progress of both mother and baby and identify any potential complications early on. Through personalized care plans and ongoing support, healthcare professionals can help mitigate risks and optimize maternal and fetal health.

6. Looking Ahead: As we embark on this journey through the complexities of pregnancy, it is essential to approach it with empathy, compassion, and a commitment to providing the best possible care for expectant mothers and their babies. By addressing the challenges head-on and fostering a supportive environment, we can help ensure that every pregnancy is a safe and fulfilling experience for all involved.

In the chapters that follow, we will explore in greater detail the specific challenges and solutions associated with various aspects of pregnancy, from prenatal nutrition and exercise to labor and delivery. Together, let us navigate the journey of pregnancy with knowledge, compassion, and a steadfast dedication to the well-being of mothers and their precious little ones.

UNDERSTANDING THE FEMALE REPRODUCTIVE SYSTEM

The female reproductive system is a marvel of biological engineering, intricately designed to facilitate the conception, development, and birth of new life. In this chapter, we will explore the anatomy and physiology of the female reproductive system, delving into its various components and functions. Understanding the intricacies of this system is essential for comprehending the processes involved in pregnancy and addressing potential problems that may arise.

1. Anatomy of the Female Reproductive System:

a. Ovaries:

- The ovaries are the primary organs of the female reproductive system responsible for producing eggs (ova) and female sex hormones, including estrogen and progesterone.

- Located on either side of the uterus, the ovaries release mature eggs during ovulation, which occurs approximately once a month during the menstrual cycle.

b. Fallopian Tubes:

- The fallopian tubes are narrow, tube-like structures that connect the ovaries to the uterus.

- Their primary function is to transport eggs from the ovaries to the uterus, where fertilization typically occurs.

c. Uterus:

- The uterus, also known as the womb, is a pear-shaped organ where fetal development takes place during pregnancy.

- It consists of three layers: the endometrium, myometrium, and perimetrium, each serving a specific function in supporting pregnancy.

d. Cervix:

- The cervix is the lower portion of the uterus that connects it to the vagina.

- It plays a crucial role in pregnancy by providing structural support to the developing fetus and regulating the flow of menstrual blood.

e. Vagina:

- The vagina is a muscular canal that extends from the cervix to the external genitalia.

- It serves as a passageway for menstrual flow, intercourse, and childbirth.

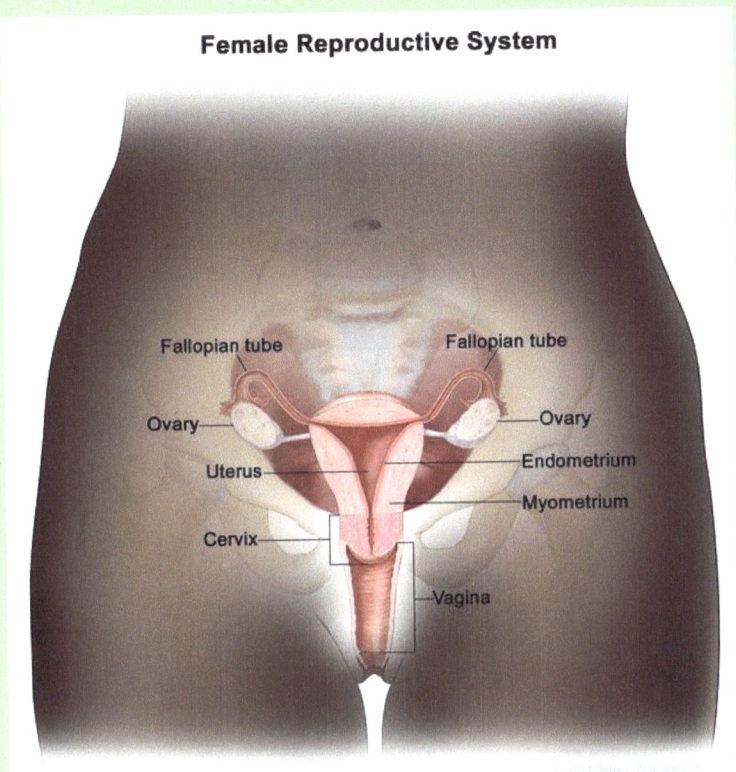

Female Reproductive System

Fallopian tube · Fallopian tube · Ovary · Ovary · Uterus · Endometrium · Myometrium · Cervix · Vagina

2. Menstrual Cycle:

a. The menstrual cycle is a series of physiological changes that occur in the female reproductive system, typically lasting around 28 days.

b. Key events of the menstrual cycle include menstruation, follicular development, ovulation, and the luteal phase.

c. Hormonal fluctuations, primarily involving estrogen and progesterone, regulate the menstrual cycle and coordinate the release of eggs from the ovaries.

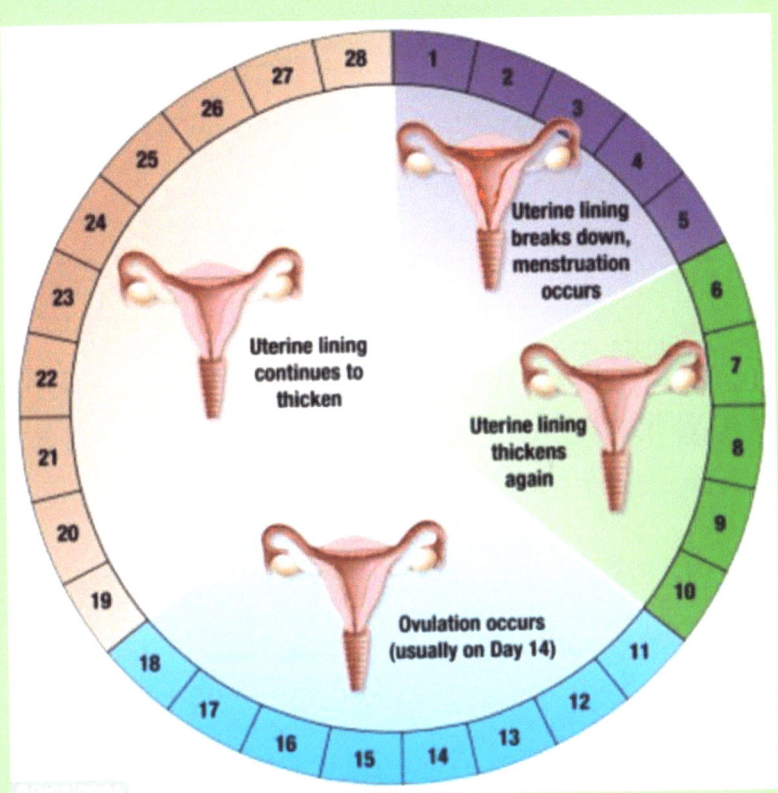

- Uterine lining breaks down, menstruation occurs
- Uterine lining thickens again
- Ovulation occurs (usually on Day 14)
- Uterine lining continues to thicken

3. Hormonal Regulation:

a. Estrogen:

- Estrogen is the primary female sex hormone responsible for the development and maintenance of female reproductive tissues.

- It plays a key role in regulating the menstrual cycle, promoting the growth of the uterine lining, and stimulating ovulation.

b. Progesterone:

- Progesterone works in conjunction with estrogen to prepare the uterus for pregnancy and support early embryonic development.

- It helps maintain the uterine lining and prevents spontaneous contractions that could disrupt pregnancy.

4. Overview of Fertilization and Implantation:

a. Fertilization occurs when a sperm cell successfully penetrates and fuses with an egg, forming a zygote.

b. The fertilized egg undergoes a series of cell divisions as it travels down the fallopian tube toward the uterus.

c. Implantation occurs when the developing embryo attaches to the uterine lining, initiating the process of pregnancy.

Conclusion:

The female reproductive system is a complex network of organs and hormones that work together to facilitate conception and support pregnancy. By understanding the anatomy and physiology of this system, we can better comprehend the processes involved in reproduction and address any issues that may arise. In the subsequent chapters, we will explore common problems and solutions related to female reproductive health,

empowering women to take control of their
reproductive well-being.

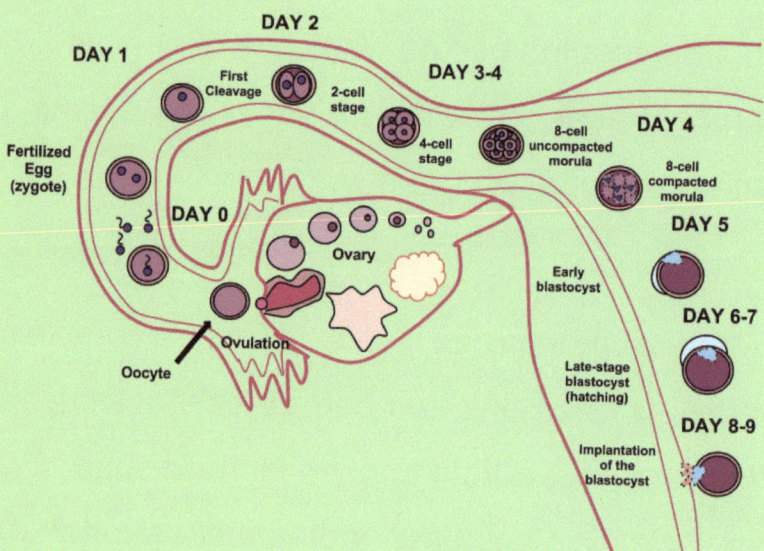

THE SCIENCE BEHIND THE PROCESS OF CONCEPTION

Introduction

Conception is the foundational event in human reproduction, marking the beginning of a new life. While it may seem like a simple process, conception involves a series of intricate biological events orchestrated by the reproductive systems of both males and females. In this chapter, we delve into the fascinating science behind conception, exploring the mechanisms that govern fertilization and early embryo development.

1. Anatomy and Physiology of Reproductive Organs

1.1 Male Reproductive System

- Overview of male reproductive anatomy

- Functions of the testes, epididymis, vas deferens, and accessory glands

- Production and maturation of spermatozoa

- Role of hormones in male reproduction: testosterone, follicle-stimulating hormone (FSH), and luteinizing hormone (LH)

1.2 Female Reproductive System

- Overview of female reproductive anatomy, including the ovaries, fallopian tubes, uterus, and vagina

- The menstrual cycle: phases and hormonal regulation

- Ovulation: release of the mature egg from the ovary

- Hormonal control by estrogen, progesterone, FSH, and LH

2. The Journey of Sperm and Egg

2.1 Spermatogenesis

- Process of sperm production in the testes

- Structure and function of sperm cells

- Factors affecting sperm health and motility

2.2 Oogenesis

- Formation and maturation of ova (eggs) in the ovaries

- Monthly ovulation cycle and release of the egg

- Factors influencing female fertility and egg quality

2.3 Fertilization

- The meeting of sperm and egg in the fallopian tube

- Sperm-egg recognition and binding

- Fusion of genetic material: formation of the zygote

3. Early Embryo Development

3.1 Cleavage and Blastocyst Formation

- Division of the fertilized egg into multiple cells

- Formation of the blastocyst: differentiation into inner cell mass and trophoblast

3.2 Implantation

- Attachment of the blastocyst to the uterine lining

- Role of hormones in facilitating implantation

- Establishment of maternal-fetal circulation

3.3 Embryogenesis

- Formation of embryonic germ layers: ectoderm, mesoderm, and endoderm

- Development of major organ systems

- Critical stages of embryonic development and potential abnormalities

Conclusion

Understanding the science behind the process of conception is essential for addressing fertility issues, optimizing reproductive health, and supporting successful pregnancies. By unraveling the intricacies of male and female reproductive biology, we gain insights into the factors influencing fertility and the potential avenues for intervention and treatment. Through ongoing research and medical advancements, we continue to expand our knowledge of conception, fostering healthier outcomes for individuals and families worldwide.

COMMON CONCEPTION/FERTILITY PROBLEMS AND CAUSES

Conceiving a child is a deeply personal and often eagerly anticipated journey for many individuals and couples. However, for some, achieving pregnancy can present challenges and obstacles that require understanding, diagnosis, and treatment. In this chapter, we explore the common conception and fertility problems faced by individuals and couples, along with their underlying causes.

1. Infertility: Definition and Prevalence

1.1 Understanding Infertility

- Defining infertility and its significance

- Differentiating between primary and secondary infertility

- Prevalence of infertility worldwide and its impact on individuals and relationships

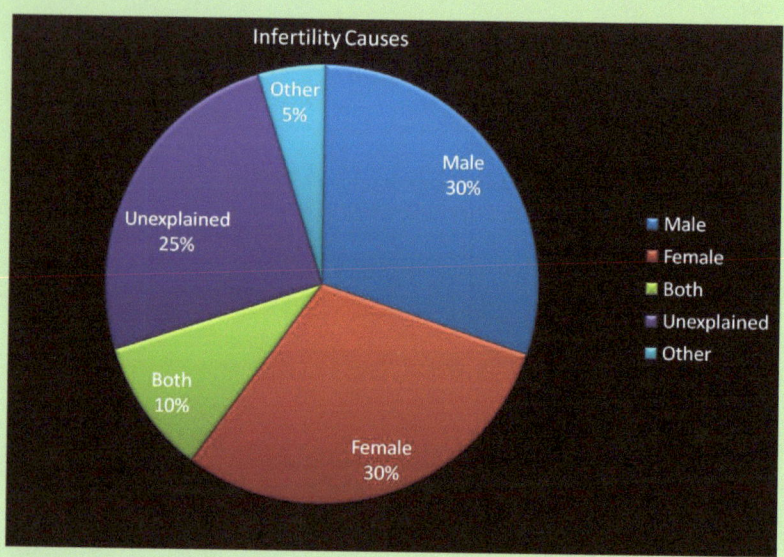

1.2 Factors Contributing to Infertility

- Age-related decline in fertility

- Lifestyle factors: diet, exercise, smoking, alcohol, and stress

- Medical conditions affecting fertility: polycystic ovary syndrome (PCOS), endometriosis, and thyroid disorders

- Genetic factors and inherited conditions

2. Ovulatory Disorders

2.1 Anovulation

- Causes of anovulation: hormonal imbalances, polycystic ovary syndrome (PCOS), and thyroid disorders

- Diagnostic methods: hormone testing, ultrasound, and ovulation tracking

- Treatment options: lifestyle modifications, medications, and assisted reproductive technologies (ART)

2.2 Irregular Menstrual Cycles

- Understanding irregular menstrual cycles and their impact on fertility

- Identifying underlying causes: hormonal imbalances, stress, and lifestyle factors

- Treatment approaches: hormone therapy, stress management, and lifestyle adjustments

3. Male Factor Infertility

3.1 Semen Analysis

- Importance of semen analysis in assessing male fertility

- Parameters evaluated: sperm count, motility, morphology, and semen volume

- Diagnostic criteria for male factor infertility

3.2 Causes of Male Factor Infertility

- Structural abnormalities: varicocele, obstructive azoospermia, and ejaculatory dysfunction

- Hormonal imbalances: low testosterone, elevated prolactin levels, and thyroid disorders

- Lifestyle factors: smoking, alcohol consumption, and exposure to toxins

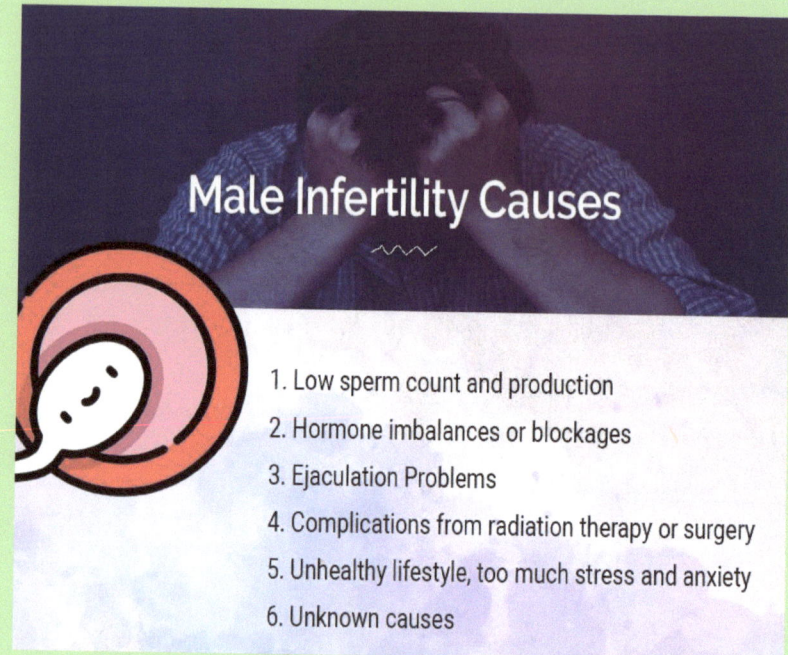

Male Infertility Causes

1. Low sperm count and production
2. Hormone imbalances or blockages
3. Ejaculation Problems
4. Complications from radiation therapy or surgery
5. Unhealthy lifestyle, too much stress and anxiety
6. Unknown causes

4. Tubal and Uterine Factors

4.1 Tubal Factors

- Understanding tubal infertility: blockages, adhesions, and tubal ligation

- Diagnostic methods: hysterosalpingography (HSG) and laparoscopy

- Treatment options: surgical interventions and assisted reproductive technologies (ART)

4.2 Uterine Factors

- Conditions affecting uterine fertility: fibroids, polyps, and uterine abnormalities

- Diagnostic evaluation: ultrasound, hysteroscopy, and MRI

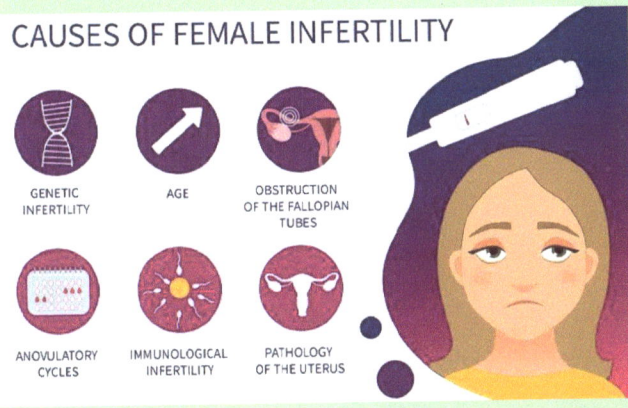

- Treatment approaches: surgical removal of abnormalities, hormonal therapy, and assisted reproductive technologies (ART)

Conclusion

Conception and fertility problems can present complex challenges for individuals and couples striving to achieve pregnancy. By understanding the common issues and underlying causes discussed in this chapter, healthcare providers can offer comprehensive evaluation, diagnosis, and tailored treatment plans to support individuals on their journey to parenthood. Through advancements in medical science and fertility treatments, many individuals facing conception challenges can find hope and solutions to realize their dreams of starting or expanding their families.

LIFESTYLE, NUTRITION, AND CONCEPTION

The journey to conception is influenced by a multitude of factors, including lifestyle choices and nutritional habits. In this chapter, we explore the intricate relationship between lifestyle, nutrition, and the process of conception. Understanding how these factors impact fertility can empower individuals and couples to make informed decisions to optimize their chances of achieving a healthy pregnancy.

1. The Impact of Lifestyle Choices on Fertility

1.1 Smoking

- Effects of smoking on male and female fertility

- Mechanisms of reproductive damage caused by smoking

- Strategies for smoking cessation to improve fertility outcomes

1.2 Alcohol Consumption

- Influence of alcohol on reproductive hormones and menstrual cycle

- Impact of alcohol on male and female fertility

- Guidelines for moderate alcohol consumption during conception attempts

1.3 Drug Use

- Risks associated with recreational drug use on fertility

- Common drugs that may impair fertility in both men and women

- Importance of seeking support for substance abuse issues when attempting conception

1.4 Stress Management

- The relationship between stress and fertility

- Physiological mechanisms linking stress to reproductive health

- Coping strategies and relaxation techniques to mitigate stress during conception attempts

2. Nutrition and Fertility

2.1 Importance of a Balanced Diet

- Nutritional requirements for optimal reproductive health

- Impact of macronutrients (carbohydrates, proteins, fats) on fertility

- Incorporating a variety of fruits, vegetables, whole grains, and lean proteins into the diet

2.2 Micronutrients and Fertility

- Role of vitamins and minerals in supporting fertility

- Essential micronutrients for male and female reproductive health: folate, zinc, vitamin D, and omega-3 fatty acids

- Dietary sources and supplementation recommendations for key micronutrients

2.3 Weight Management

- The relationship between body weight and fertility

- Effects of obesity and underweight on reproductive hormones and menstrual cycle

- Strategies for achieving and maintaining a healthy weight for fertility optimization

3. Physical Activity and Fertility

3.1 Benefits of Exercise

- Impact of regular physical activity on fertility

- Effects of exercise on reproductive hormones and menstrual cycle regularity

- Guidelines for safe and effective exercise during conception attempts

3.2 Avoidance of Overexertion

- Risks associated with excessive exercise and fertility

- Finding a balance between physical activity and rest for fertility optimization

- Consulting with healthcare providers for personalized exercise recommendations

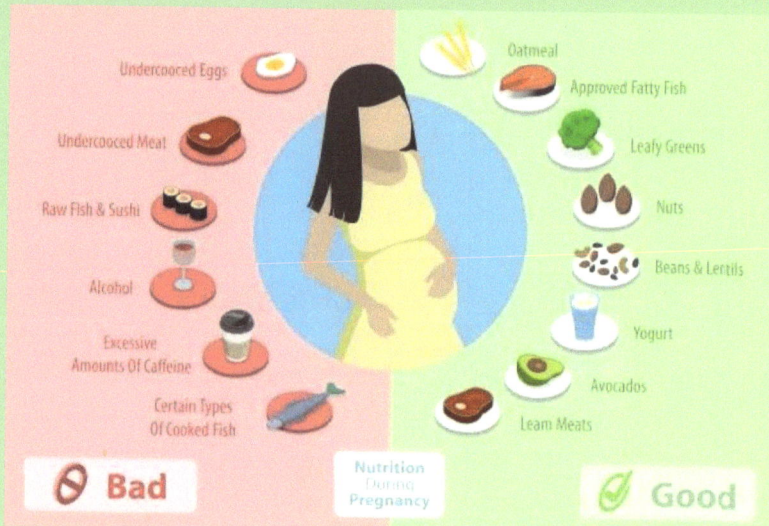

Conclusion

Lifestyle choices and nutritional habits play a significant role in shaping reproductive health and fertility outcomes. By adopting healthy lifestyle practices, including smoking cessation, moderation in alcohol consumption, stress management, balanced nutrition, and regular physical activity, individuals and couples can enhance their chances of conceiving and experiencing a healthy pregnancy. Through informed decision-making and proactive measures, individuals can take charge of their reproductive journey and pave the way for a successful conception and pregnancy.

WOMEN'S HEALTH AND CONCEPTION

Introduction

Women's health is intricately linked to the process of conception, pregnancy, and childbirth. In this chapter, we delve into the various aspects of women's health that can impact conception, from reproductive disorders to general well-being. By understanding and addressing women's health concerns, individuals and couples can optimize their fertility and enhance their chances of achieving a healthy pregnancy.

1. Reproductive Health Assessment

1.1 Menstrual Health

- Importance of regular menstrual cycles for fertility

- Common menstrual disorders: amenorrhea, oligomenorrhea, and irregular cycles

- Evaluation and management of menstrual irregularities in the context of conception

1.2 Hormonal Imbalances

- Role of hormones in regulating the menstrual cycle and ovulation

- Common hormonal disorders affecting fertility: polycystic ovary syndrome (PCOS), thyroid disorders, and hyperprolactinemia

- Diagnostic evaluation and treatment approaches for hormonal imbalances

1.3 Pelvic Health

- Assessment of pelvic anatomy and function

- Screening for pelvic inflammatory disease (PID) and sexually transmitted infections (STIs)

- Management of pelvic conditions that may impact fertility, such as endometriosis and pelvic adhesions

2. Reproductive Disorders

2.1 Polycystic Ovary Syndrome (PCOS)

- Overview of PCOS and its impact on fertility

- Diagnostic criteria and evaluation of PCOS

- Treatment strategies to manage PCOS-related infertility

2.2 Endometriosis

- Understanding endometriosis and its effects on fertility

- Diagnosis and staging of endometriosis

- Surgical and medical management options for endometriosis-associated infertility

2.3 Uterine Fibroids

- Characteristics and prevalence of uterine fibroids

- Impact of fibroids on fertility and pregnancy outcomes

- Treatment approaches for fibroids in the context of conception

3. Preconception Care

3.1 Importance of Preconception Health

- Benefits of optimizing health before conception

- Preconception counseling and screening recommendations

- Lifestyle modifications and preventive measures for promoting a healthy pregnancy

3.2 Folic Acid Supplementation

- Role of folic acid in preventing neural tube defects

- Recommended dosage and timing of folic acid supplementation

- Incorporating folic acid into preconception care guidelines

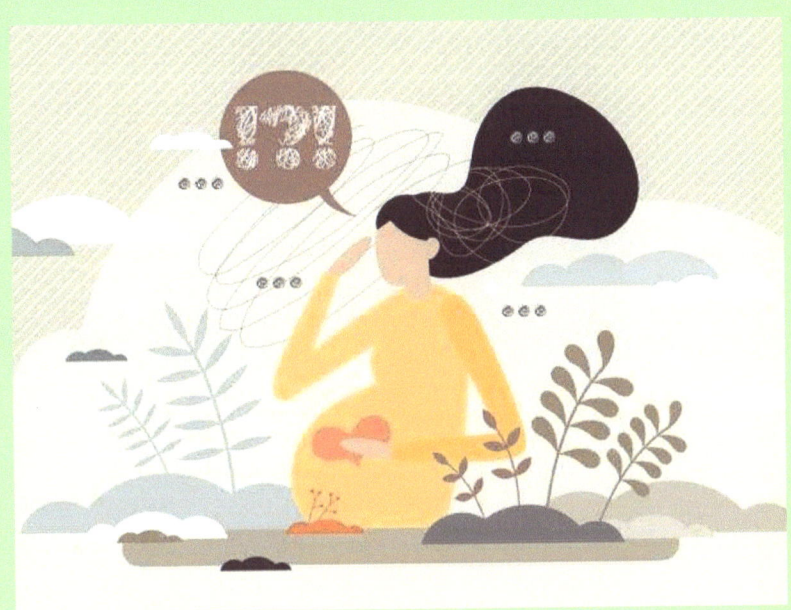

Conclusion

Women's health plays a crucial role in the journey to conception and pregnancy. By addressing reproductive health concerns, hormonal imbalances, and reproductive disorders, individuals can optimize their fertility and improve their chances of conceiving a healthy baby. Through comprehensive preconception care and proactive management of women's health issues, healthcare providers can support individuals and couples in achieving their dreams of starting or expanding their families.

MEN'S HEALTH AND CONCEPTION

While the focus of conception often centers on women's health, it is equally important to recognize the role of men's health in the process of achieving pregnancy. In this chapter, we explore various aspects of men's health that can impact fertility and conception. By understanding and addressing men's health concerns, individuals and couples can enhance their chances of successful conception and parenthood.

1. Understanding Male Fertility

1.1 Sperm Production and Function

- Anatomy of the male reproductive system

- Process of spermatogenesis: production and maturation of sperm cells

- Role of sperm in fertilization and embryo development

1.2 Factors Influencing Male Fertility

- Lifestyle factors affecting sperm quality and quantity: smoking, alcohol, and drug use

- Environmental exposures and occupational hazards

- Medical conditions impacting male fertility: varicocele, hormonal imbalances, and genetic factors

1.3 Diagnostic Evaluation of Male Fertility

- Semen analysis: assessing sperm count, motility, morphology, and other parameters

- Hormonal testing to evaluate reproductive hormone levels

- Imaging studies and genetic testing when indicated

2. Lifestyle Modifications for Improved Fertility

2.1 Smoking Cessation

- Effects of smoking on sperm quality and fertility

- Benefits of quitting smoking for male reproductive health

- Support resources and strategies for smoking cessation

2.2 Alcohol and Substance Use

- Impact of alcohol consumption and recreational drug use on male fertility

- Guidelines for moderate alcohol consumption and avoidance of substance abuse

- Seeking help for substance abuse issues and addiction recovery

2.3 Diet and Nutrition

- Importance of a balanced diet for optimal sperm production and function

- Nutrients essential for male fertility: zinc, folate, antioxidants, and omega-3 fatty acids

- Dietary recommendations for promoting reproductive health

3. Managing Medical Conditions Affecting Male Fertility

3.1 Varicocele

- Definition and prevalence of varicocele

- Effects of varicocele on sperm production and testicular function

- Treatment options: surgical repair and minimally invasive procedures

3.2 Hormonal Imbalances

- Common hormonal disorders affecting male fertility: hypogonadism and hyperprolactinemia

- Diagnostic evaluation and treatment approaches for hormonal imbalances

- Hormone replacement therapy and other interventions to restore fertility

3.3 Genetic Factors

- Inherited conditions impacting male fertility: Klinefelter syndrome, Y chromosome microdeletions, and chromosomal abnormalities

- Genetic counseling and testing for couples with a family history of genetic disorders

- Assisted reproductive technologies (ART) for overcoming genetic infertility

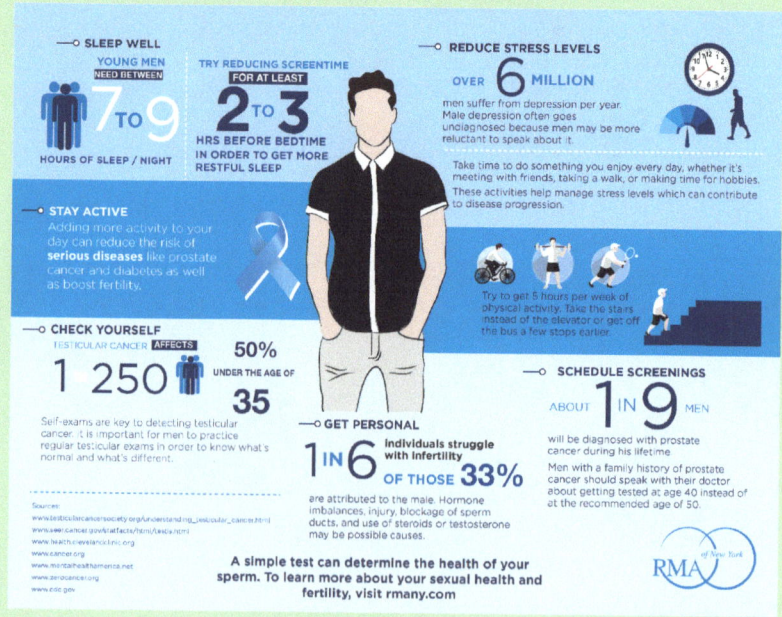

Conclusion

Men's health plays a critical role in the journey to conception and parenthood. By addressing lifestyle factors, managing medical conditions, and seeking appropriate care for male fertility issues, individuals can enhance their reproductive health and contribute to successful conception outcomes. Through awareness, proactive health management, and collaborative care, men can play an active role in achieving their goals of starting or expanding their families.

MENTAL HEALTH AND CONCEPTION

Mental health plays a crucial role in every aspect of our lives, including the process of conception. The mind-body connection has been increasingly recognized in reproductive health, and research indicates that mental well-being can significantly impact fertility and conception. In this chapter, we will explore the intricate relationship between mental health and conception, discussing the various psychological factors that can influence fertility and providing strategies and solutions for maintaining optimal mental well-being during the conception journey.

Understanding the Mind-Body Connection

The mind and body are intricately connected, and this connection extends to the realm of reproductive health. Research has shown that stress, anxiety, depression, and other mental health issues can impact fertility by disrupting hormonal balance, menstrual cycles, and overall reproductive function. Moreover, the stress associated with fertility struggles can create a vicious cycle, further exacerbating psychological distress and affecting fertility outcomes.

Managing Stress and Anxiety

Stress and anxiety are common experiences for individuals navigating the conception journey, whether they are trying to conceive naturally or undergoing fertility treatments. It's essential to develop effective stress management techniques to mitigate the negative impact of stress on fertility. Techniques such as mindfulness meditation, deep breathing exercises, yoga, and progressive muscle relaxation can help alleviate stress and promote a sense of calm and balance.

Coping with Fertility Struggles

Dealing with fertility struggles can be emotionally challenging, leading to feelings of grief, frustration, and inadequacy. It's crucial for individuals and couples facing fertility challenges to seek support from loved ones, mental health professionals, and support groups specializing in infertility. Processing emotions, sharing experiences, and seeking professional guidance can help individuals cope more effectively with the emotional toll of fertility struggles and maintain mental well-being throughout the conception journey.

Addressing Relationship Dynamics

The process of trying to conceive can place strain on relationships, as couples navigate the emotional rollercoaster of fertility struggles, medical interventions, and uncertainty about the future. Open communication, empathy, and mutual support are essential for maintaining healthy relationships during the conception journey. Couples may benefit from couples therapy or relationship counseling to address communication barriers, strengthen emotional bonds, and navigate the challenges of infertility as a team.

Seeking Professional Help

If stress, anxiety, or depression significantly impact daily functioning or interfere with the conception journey, it's essential to seek professional help from a mental health specialist. Therapy, counseling, and psychiatric interventions can provide individuals with the support and tools they need to manage their mental health effectively and enhance fertility outcomes. Additionally, addressing underlying mental health issues can improve overall well-being and quality of life.

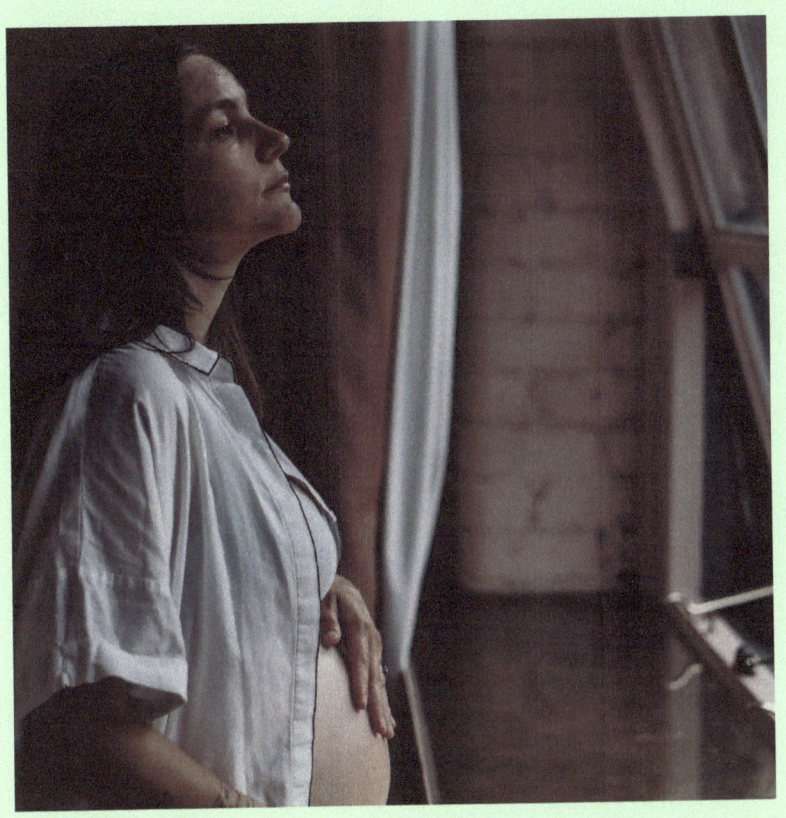

Conclusion

Mental health plays a significant role in the process of conception, influencing fertility outcomes and overall well-being. By recognizing the impact of psychological factors on fertility and implementing strategies to promote mental well-being, individuals and couples can enhance their chances of conceiving and navigate the conception journey with resilience and optimism. Remember, prioritizing self-care, seeking support, and addressing mental health needs are essential steps towards achieving a healthy conception and pregnancy.

MEDICAL EVALUATION, DIAGNOSTIC TESTS, AND PROCEDURES

A comprehensive medical evaluation, including diagnostic tests and procedures, is essential for ensuring a healthy pregnancy and addressing any potential concerns or complications. In this chapter, we will discuss the importance of medical evaluation before and during pregnancy, the various diagnostic tests and procedures available, and how they help identify and manage pregnancy-related problems.

Preconception Medical Evaluation

Before attempting to conceive, individuals should undergo a preconception medical evaluation to assess their overall health and identify any potential risk factors that may affect pregnancy. This evaluation typically includes a review of medical history, lifestyle factors, medications, immunization status, and screening for pre-existing medical conditions such as diabetes, hypertension, or thyroid disorders. Addressing any underlying health issues before conception can help optimize pregnancy outcomes and reduce the risk of complications.

Diagnostic Tests and Screening Procedures

During pregnancy, various diagnostic tests and screening procedures are performed to monitor fetal development, assess maternal health, and detect any potential problems or abnormalities. These tests may include:

1. Ultrasound: Ultrasound imaging is commonly used during pregnancy to visualize the fetus, monitor growth and development,

and assess for any structural abnormalities or anomalies

2. Maternal blood tests: Blood tests are routinely performed during pregnancy to screen for conditions such as anemia, gestational diabetes, Rh factor compatibility, and infections such as HIV, syphilis, and hepatitis.

3. Genetic screening: Genetic screening tests, such as carrier screening and non-invasive prenatal testing (NIPT), are offered to assess the risk of genetic disorders and chromosomal abnormalities, such as Down syndrome, in the fetus.

4. Amniocentesis and chorionic villus sampling (CVS): In cases where there is an increased risk of genetic abnormalities, invasive procedures such as amniocentesis

and CVS may be recommended to obtain fetal cells for further genetic analysis.

5. Non-stress test (NST) and biophysical profile (BPP): These tests are performed to assess fetal well-being and monitor fetal heart rate, movement, and breathing patterns.

6. Glucose tolerance test (GTT): This test is used to diagnose gestational diabetes by measuring blood sugar levels after consuming a glucose solution.

Managing Pregnancy-Related Problems

In addition to diagnostic tests and screening procedures, medical evaluation during pregnancy involves monitoring for and managing pregnancy-related problems and complications. This may include conditions such as preeclampsia, gestational hypertension, placental abnormalities, preterm labor, and fetal growth restriction. Early detection and prompt management of these issues are crucial for optimizing maternal and fetal outcomes.

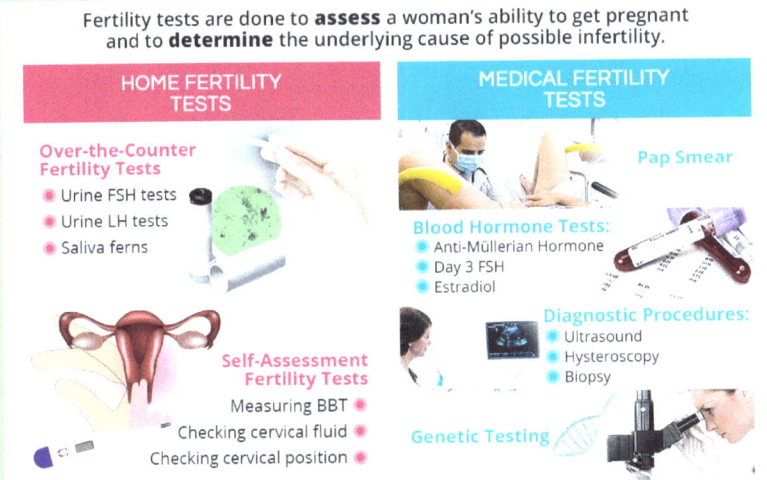

Fertility tests are done to **assess** a woman's ability to get pregnant and to **determine** the underlying cause of possible infertility.

HOME FERTILITY TESTS

Over-the-Counter Fertility Tests
- Urine FSH tests
- Urine LH tests
- Saliva ferns

Self-Assessment Fertility Tests
- Measuring BBT
- Checking cervical fluid
- Checking cervical position

MEDICAL FERTILITY TESTS

Pap Smear

Blood Hormone Tests:
- Anti-Müllerian Hormone
- Day 3 FSH
- Estradiol

Diagnostic Procedures:
- Ultrasound
- Hysteroscopy
- Biopsy

Genetic Testing

Conclusion

A thorough medical evaluation, including diagnostic tests and procedures, is essential for ensuring a healthy pregnancy and addressing any potential problems or complications. By identifying risk factors, monitoring fetal development, and managing pregnancy-related issues, healthcare providers can help individuals achieve a safe and successful pregnancy. It's important for individuals to actively participate in their prenatal care, communicate any concerns with their healthcare provider, and follow recommended screening and monitoring protocols to promote the best possible outcomes for themselves and their babies.

INTERVENTIONS AND TREATMENTS: MEDICAL, LIFESTYLE, AND SURGICAL

Navigating pregnancy involves a myriad of considerations, including interventions and treatments aimed at ensuring the health and well-being of both the mother and the developing fetus. In this chapter, we will explore various medical, lifestyle, and surgical interventions commonly employed to address pregnancy-related issues and optimize maternal and fetal outcomes.

Medical Interventions

1. Prenatal Vitamins: Prenatal vitamins containing folic acid, iron, calcium, and other essential nutrients are recommended for all

pregnant individuals to support maternal health and fetal development.

2. Medications: In some cases, medications may be prescribed during pregnancy to manage specific conditions such as gestational diabetes, hypertension, thyroid disorders, or infections. It's essential to consult with a healthcare provider before taking any medication during pregnancy to ensure safety for both the mother and the baby.

3. Antenatal Testing: Antenatal testing, including ultrasounds, fetal monitoring, and genetic screening, is routinely performed to monitor fetal growth and development, assess fetal well-being, and detect any potential problems or abnormalities.

4. Tocolytic Therapy: Tocolytic medications may be used to suppress uterine contractions and prevent preterm labor in individuals at risk of delivering prematurely.

Lifestyle Interventions

1. Nutrition and Diet: A balanced and nutritious diet is crucial during pregnancy to support maternal health and fetal development. Pregnant individuals should aim to consume a variety of nutrient-rich foods, including fruits, vegetables, lean proteins, whole grains, and dairy products, while avoiding excessive caffeine, alcohol, and processed foods.

2. Exercise: Regular physical activity during pregnancy can provide numerous benefits, including improved cardiovascular health, reduced risk of gestational diabetes and

preeclampsia, and enhanced mood and well-being. Pregnant individuals should consult with their healthcare provider before starting or modifying an exercise regimen and aim for activities that are safe and appropriate for their stage of pregnancy.

3. Smoking Cessation: Smoking during pregnancy is associated with numerous adverse outcomes, including preterm birth, low birth weight, and birth defects. Pregnant individuals who smoke should quit smoking to improve their health and reduce the risk of complications for themselves and their babies.

Surgical Interventions

1. Cesarean Section: A cesarean section (C-section) may be recommended in cases where vaginal delivery poses risks to the mother or the baby, such as placenta previa,

fetal distress, or prior uterine surgery. Cesarean sections are also performed electively in certain situations, such as breech presentation or multiple pregnancies.

2. Surgical Management of Pregnancy Complications: Surgical interventions may be necessary to manage pregnancy complications such as ectopic pregnancy, placental abnormalities, or fetal anomalies. These procedures are performed by obstetricians and other specialized healthcare providers to optimize maternal and fetal outcomes.

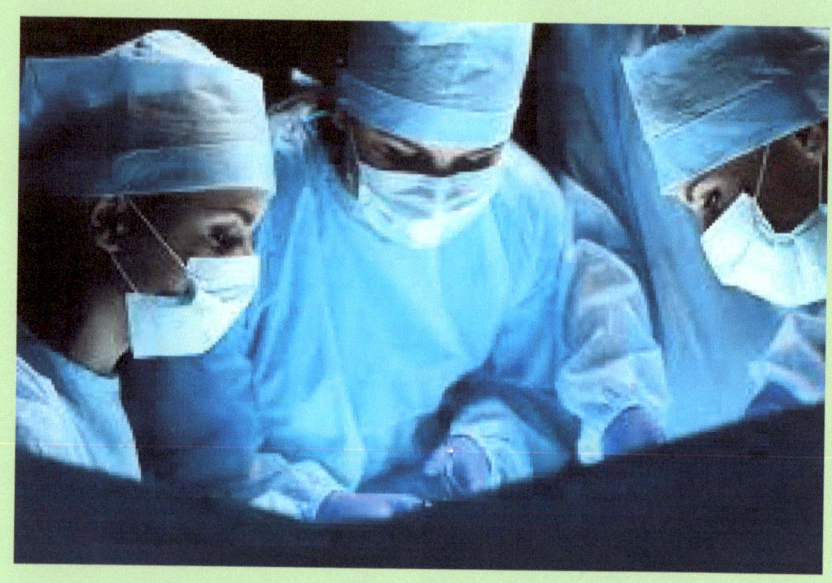

Conclusion

Interventions and treatments play a critical role in ensuring the health and well-being of both the mother and the developing fetus during pregnancy. Whether medical, lifestyle, or surgical in nature, these interventions are aimed at addressing pregnancy-related issues, managing complications, and promoting optimal maternal and fetal outcomes. It's essential for pregnant individuals to work closely with their healthcare providers to develop personalized treatment plans that prioritize safety and effectiveness for both themselves and their babies.

ALTERNATIVE THERAPIES AND HOLISTIC APPROACHES

In recent years, there has been growing interest in alternative therapies and holistic approaches to pregnancy care, complementing traditional medical interventions. These approaches aim to promote maternal well-being, support natural birthing processes, and enhance the overall pregnancy experience. In this chapter, we will explore various alternative therapies and holistic approaches commonly utilized during pregnancy, discussing their benefits, safety considerations, and potential roles in optimizing maternal and fetal outcomes.

1. Acupuncture and Acupressure

Acupuncture and acupressure involve the stimulation of specific points on the body to promote balance and alleviate various symptoms. During pregnancy, acupuncture and acupressure may be used to relieve nausea and vomiting, alleviate back pain, reduce anxiety, and facilitate labor induction. These techniques are generally considered safe when performed by trained practitioners but should be used with caution in certain pregnancy conditions and always under the guidance of a qualified healthcare provider.

2. Chiropractic Care

Chiropractic care focuses on the alignment of the spine and musculoskeletal system to promote overall health and well-being. Pregnant individuals may seek chiropractic care to alleviate back pain, pelvic discomfort, and other musculoskeletal issues associated with pregnancy. Chiropractic adjustments during pregnancy should be performed by practitioners with specialized training in prenatal care and are generally considered safe and effective for most pregnant individuals.

3. Massage Therapy

Massage therapy offers numerous benefits during pregnancy, including stress reduction, pain relief, improved circulation, and relaxation. Prenatal massage techniques are specifically tailored to accommodate the unique needs and comfort of pregnant individuals, focusing on areas of tension and discomfort. Massage therapy during pregnancy should be performed by certified prenatal massage therapists who are trained to provide safe and appropriate care for pregnant clients.

4. Yoga and Meditation

Yoga and meditation practices can be valuable tools for promoting physical and mental well-being during pregnancy. Prenatal yoga classes offer gentle stretches, strengthening exercises, and relaxation techniques designed to support the changing needs of pregnant bodies and prepare individuals for childbirth. Similarly, meditation and mindfulness practices can help reduce stress, anxiety, and discomfort during pregnancy, promoting a sense of calm and inner peace.

5. Herbal Remedies and Aromatherapy

Herbal remedies and aromatherapy involve the use of plant-based products and essential oils to address various pregnancy-related symptoms and promote overall wellness. While some herbal remedies and essential oils are considered safe during pregnancy when used in moderation and under the guidance of a qualified herbalist or aromatherapist, others may pose risks to maternal and fetal health and should be avoided. Pregnant individuals should exercise caution and consult with their healthcare provider before using any herbal remedies or essential oils during pregnancy.

Conclusion

Alternative therapies and holistic approaches can complement traditional medical interventions and enhance the overall pregnancy experience by promoting maternal well-being, supporting natural birthing processes, and addressing pregnancy-related symptoms. However, it's essential for pregnant individuals to approach these therapies with caution, seek guidance from qualified practitioners, and communicate openly with their healthcare providers about their use of alternative therapies during pregnancy. By incorporating a holistic approach to pregnancy care, individuals can cultivate a sense of balance, empowerment, and connection throughout the journey to motherhood.

MODERN TECHNOLOGICAL SOLUTIONS: ASSISTED REPRODUCTIVE TECHNOLOGIES (ART)

Advancements in medical science have revolutionized the field of reproductive medicine, offering hope to individuals and couples facing challenges with conception. Assisted Reproductive Technologies (ART) encompass a range of innovative procedures and techniques designed to overcome fertility obstacles and facilitate conception. In this chapter, we will explore various ART options, their applications, success rates, and ethical considerations, providing insight into the modern technological solutions available to individuals seeking to build their families.

1. In vitro Fertilization (IVF)

In vitro fertilization (IVF) is one of the most widely known and commonly performed ART procedures. It involves the retrieval of eggs from the ovaries, fertilization with sperm in a laboratory setting, and the transfer of resulting embryos into the uterus. IVF may be recommended for individuals or couples with infertility due to factors such as tubal blockage, male factor infertility, ovulatory disorders, or unexplained infertility. Success rates of IVF vary depending on factors such as age, underlying fertility issues, and the quality of embryos transferred.

2. Intracytoplasmic Sperm Injection (ICSI)

Intracytoplasmic sperm injection (ICSI) is a specialized form of IVF that involves the direct injection of a single sperm into an egg to facilitate fertilization. ICSI is commonly used in cases of male factor infertility, such as low sperm count, poor sperm motility, or abnormal sperm morphology. This technique bypasses natural barriers to fertilization and can significantly improve the chances of successful conception in couples facing male infertility issues.

3. Assisted Hatching

Assisted hatching is a laboratory technique used to enhance the implantation potential of embryos during IVF. It involves creating a small opening in the outer shell (zona pellucida) of the embryo to facilitate embryo hatching and implantation in the uterine lining. Assisted hatching may be recommended for individuals or couples with a history of failed IVF cycles or advanced maternal age, as it can improve embryo implantation rates and increase the likelihood of successful pregnancy.

4. Preimplantation Genetic Testing (PGT)

Preimplantation genetic testing (PGT) involves the screening of embryos for genetic abnormalities before transfer during IVF. PGT can identify chromosomal abnormalities, single gene disorders, or structural rearrangements in embryos, allowing for the selection of genetically normal embryos for transfer. This technology can help reduce the risk of genetic disorders and miscarriage and improve the chances of a successful pregnancy for individuals or couples with a known genetic risk or recurrent pregnancy loss.

5. Cryopreservation

Cryopreservation, or embryo freezing, allows for the storage of excess embryos created during IVF for future use. Cryopreserved embryos can be thawed and transferred in subsequent IVF cycles, offering individuals or couples the opportunity to pursue pregnancy without the need for additional ovarian stimulation or egg retrieval procedures. Cryopreservation also allows for the preservation of fertility for individuals undergoing medical treatments that may impact fertility, such as chemotherapy or radiation therapy.

Ethical Considerations and Future Directions

While ART has revolutionized fertility treatment and helped millions of individuals achieve their dream of parenthood, it also raises important ethical considerations regarding the use of technology to create and manipulate human life. Key ethical issues in ART include concerns about the safety and welfare of individuals involved, the commodification of human gametes and embryos, and the social implications of assisted reproduction. As ART continues to evolve, ongoing dialogue and ethical reflection are essential to ensure that technological advancements are used responsibly and ethically to support the well-being of individuals and families.

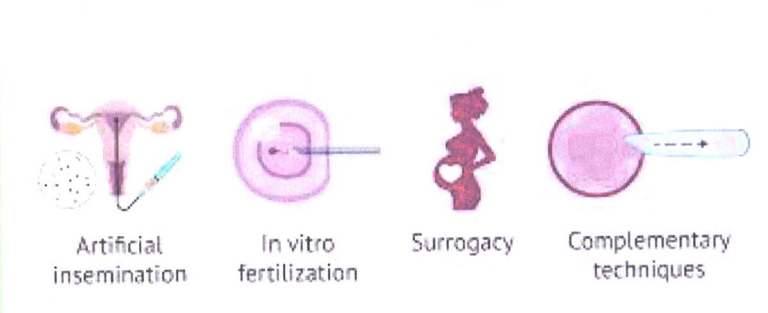

| Artificial insemination | In vitro fertilization | Surrogacy | Complementary techniques |

Conclusion

Assisted Reproductive Technologies (ART) offer modern technological solutions to individuals and couples facing challenges with conception, providing hope and opportunities for building families. From in vitro fertilization (IVF) to preimplantation genetic testing (PGT), these innovative procedures and techniques have revolutionized the field of reproductive medicine, enabling millions of individuals worldwide to achieve their dream of parenthood. As ART continues to advance, it is essential to balance technological innovation with ethical considerations, ensuring that fertility treatments are safe, effective, and ethically responsible. By harnessing the power of modern technology and scientific advancements, individuals and couples can overcome fertility obstacles and embark on the journey to parenthood with confidence and optimism.

EMOTIONAL AND PSYCHOLOGICAL SUPPORT FOR COUPLES FACING

CHALLENGES AND STRESS DURING PREGNANCY

Pregnancy is a time of profound emotional and psychological significance for couples, marked by anticipation, joy, and sometimes, challenges and stress. Navigating the complexities of pregnancy-related issues can take a toll on couples' emotional well-being, highlighting the importance of emotional and psychological support throughout the journey. In this chapter, we will explore the unique emotional and psychological challenges faced by couples during pregnancy, and discuss strategies and resources for providing effective support and coping mechanisms. Understanding Emotional and Psychological Challenges

Couples facing pregnancy-related challenges may experience a range of emotions, including anxiety, fear, frustration, sadness, and uncertainty. Common stressors may include fertility struggles, pregnancy complications, prenatal diagnosis of genetic conditions, financial concerns, relationship dynamics, and the transition to parenthood. It's essential to recognize and validate these emotions, as they are a natural response to the challenges and uncertainties of pregnancy.

Effective Coping Strategies

1. Open Communication: Honest and open communication is essential for couples facing pregnancy-related challenges. Encourage couples to express their thoughts, feelings, and concerns with each other in a safe and

supportive environment. Active listening, empathy, and validation can help strengthen emotional bonds and foster a sense of connection and understanding.

2. Seeking Support: Encourage couples to seek support from family, friends, support groups, and mental health professionals specializing in reproductive health. Sharing experiences, seeking guidance, and receiving emotional support from others who have walked a similar path can provide validation, reassurance, and a sense of community.

3. Self-Care Practices: Encourage couples to prioritize self-care practices to manage stress and promote emotional well-being. This may include engaging in activities they enjoy, practicing relaxation techniques such as mindfulness meditation or yoga, getting

regular exercise, maintaining a healthy diet, and ensuring adequate sleep.

4. Professional Counseling: Couples may benefit from professional counseling or therapy to address emotional and psychological challenges related to pregnancy. Counseling can provide a safe and confidential space to explore feelings, develop coping strategies, improve communication skills, and strengthen the couple's relationship.

5. Education and Information: Provide couples with accurate and reliable information about pregnancy-related issues, treatment options, and resources available to them. Knowledge empowers couples to make informed decisions, reduces uncertainty and anxiety,

and helps them navigate the challenges of pregnancy with confidence and resilience.

Conclusion

Emotional and psychological support is essential for couples facing challenges and stress during pregnancy. By recognizing and validating their emotions, fostering open communication, seeking support, practicing self-care, and accessing professional counseling when needed, couples can navigate the complexities of pregnancy with resilience and strength. As healthcare providers, it's crucial to offer compassionate and holistic care that addresses the emotional and psychological needs of couples, promoting their well-being and enhancing their pregnancy experience. By working together as a supportive team, couples can overcome challenges, strengthen their relationship, and embrace the journey to parenthood with confidence and optimism.

_____

ALTERNATE OPTIONS TO BECOME PARENTS

While traditional conception methods may not always be feasible for individuals or couples, there exist alternate options that provide pathways to parenthood. In this chapter, we will explore various alternative options for individuals and couples who are seeking to become parents, including adoption, surrogacy, fostering, and other non-traditional avenues.

1. Adoption

Adoption is a legal process that allows individuals or couples to become parents to a child who is not biologically related to them. There are various types of adoption, including domestic adoption, international adoption, and foster care adoption. Adoption offers a fulfilling and rewarding way to build a family and provides a loving home to children in need. Prospective adoptive parents undergo a thorough screening process and may work with adoption agencies, attorneys, or facilitators to navigate the adoption process.

2. Surrogacy

Surrogacy involves a woman (the surrogate) carrying and delivering a baby on behalf of intended parents. There are two main types of surrogacy: traditional surrogacy, where the surrogate's own egg is fertilized with sperm from the intended father or a donor, and gestational surrogacy, where the surrogate carries an embryo created using the intended parents' or donors' gametes. Surrogacy can be a complex and expensive process, involving legal agreements, medical procedures, and emotional considerations, but it provides a viable option for individuals or couples who are unable to carry a pregnancy themselves.

3. Fostering

Fostering involves providing temporary care and support to children who are unable to live with their birth families due to various reasons, such as neglect, abuse, or parental incarceration. Foster parents play a crucial role in providing stability, love, and nurturing to children during challenging times and may eventually pursue adoption if reunification with the birth family is not possible. Fostering offers an opportunity to make a positive impact on a child's life and provides a supportive environment for children in need of care and protection.

4. Donor Gametes

Donor gametes, including sperm, eggs, or embryos, can be used to facilitate conception for individuals or couples experiencing infertility or genetic concerns. Donor gametes may be obtained from known donors, such as family members or friends, or anonymous donors through fertility clinics or donor agencies. Donor gametes offer a way to overcome biological barriers to conception and enable individuals or couples to achieve their dream of parenthood.

Conclusion

Alternate options to become parents offer viable pathways to individuals or couples who are unable to conceive or carry a pregnancy themselves. Whether through adoption, surrogacy, fostering, or the use of donor gametes, these alternative options provide opportunities to build loving and nurturing families, fulfilling the desire for parenthood and enriching the lives of both parents and children. It's essential for individuals or couples considering alternate options to thoroughly research and consider their options, seek guidance from professionals, and make informed decisions that align with their values, preferences, and circumstances. By exploring alternate options with an open mind and heart, individuals or couples can embark on the journey to parenthood with hope, resilience, and joy.

CONCLUSION: EMPOWERMENT AND HOPE

As we conclude our exploration of pregnancy-related challenges and solutions, it's important to reflect on the overarching themes of empowerment and hope that permeate the journey to parenthood. Throughout this book, we have delved into various aspects of pregnancy, including medical interventions, emotional support, alternative options, and holistic approaches, all aimed at empowering individuals and couples to navigate the complexities of pregnancy with resilience, confidence, and hope.

Empowerment Through Knowledge

Knowledge is a powerful tool that empowers individuals to make informed decisions about their health and well-being. By providing accurate and reliable information about pregnancy-related issues, treatment options, and available resources, healthcare providers empower individuals and couples to take an active role in their prenatal care, advocate for their needs, and make choices that align with their values and preferences.

Embracing Challenges with Resilience Pregnancy may present a myriad of challenges, including fertility struggles, pregnancy complications, emotional distress, and uncertainty about the future. However, it's essential to approach these challenges with resilience, strength, and determination. By acknowledging and validating their emotions, seeking support from loved ones and professionals, and adopting effective coping strategies, individuals and couples can overcome obstacles and emerge stronger and more resilient on the journey to parenthood.

Fostering Hope for the Future

Hope is a powerful force that sustains us through difficult times and fuels our aspirations for the future. Despite the uncertainties and setbacks that may arise during pregnancy, it's important to maintain hope and optimism for the possibilities that lie ahead. Whether through medical interventions, alternative options, emotional support, or holistic approaches, there are countless pathways to parenthood, each offering opportunities for growth, fulfillment, and joy.

Conclusion

As we conclude our exploration of pregnancy problems and solutions, let us remember that the journey to parenthood is a deeply personal and transformative experience, marked by challenges, triumphs, and profound moments of love and connection. By empowering individuals and couples with knowledge, supporting them with compassion and empathy, and fostering hope for the future, we can help them navigate the complexities of pregnancy with confidence, resilience, and optimism. As healthcare providers, let us continue to stand alongside individuals and couples on their journey to parenthood, offering guidance, support, and encouragement every step of the way. Together, let us embrace the power of empowerment and hope as we embark on the extraordinary adventure of creating and nurturing new life.

www.ingramcontent.com/pod-product-compliance
Lightning Source LLC
Chambersburg PA
CBHW040757240526
45474CB00008B/88